Essential Heroes and Mike Melaleuca

By Caleb Selby

Illustrated by Fenny Fu

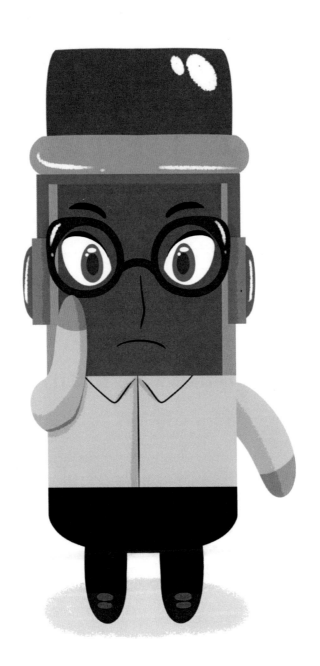

This is Mike Melaleuca!

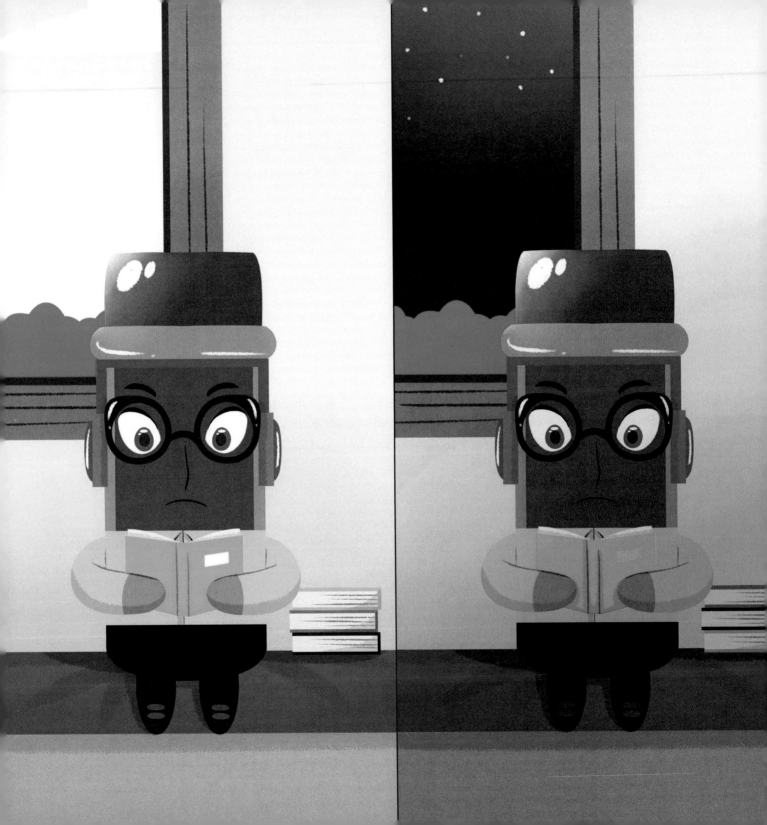

Mike Melaleuca is serious, determined and smart! The one thing Mike likes to do more than anything else is read. He reads books from morning to night. His favorite books are adventure ones, but he loves mystery and action books too!

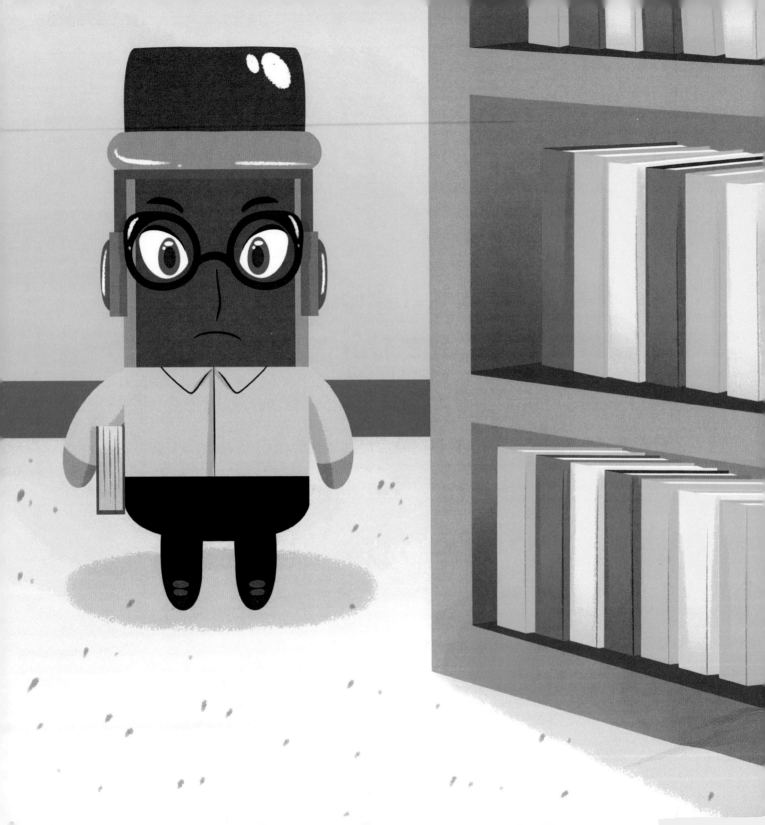

When Mike is not home reading an exciting book, he spends time at the local Bodyville library looking for interesting new stories.

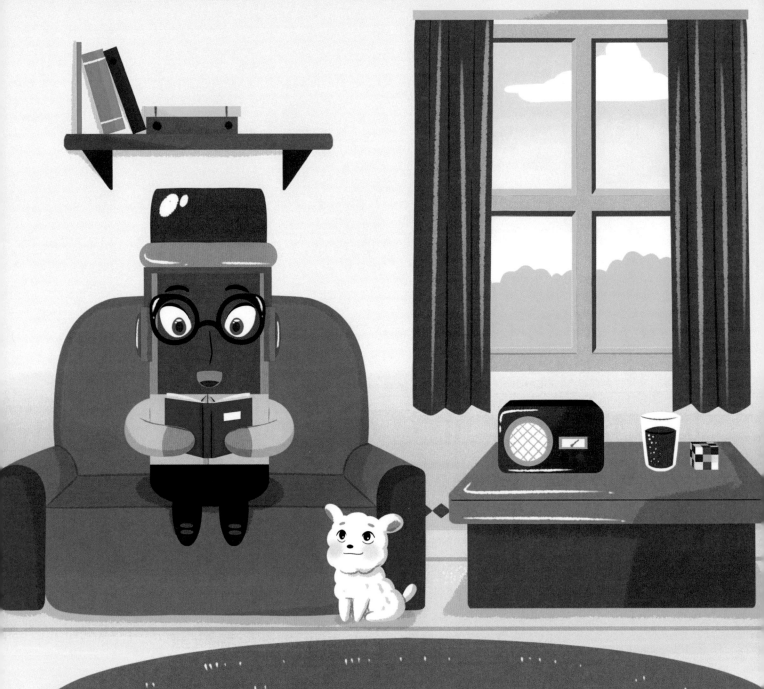

Mike likes to read his favorite books to his pet puppy named, Charlie. Mike and Charlie are best friends and they live in a little house not too far from the library. On nice days, the two of them walk to the library together and pick out books.

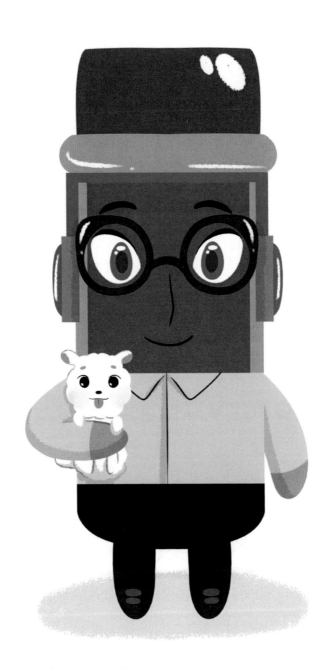

Mike is well liked by all his friends and neighbors in Bodyville.

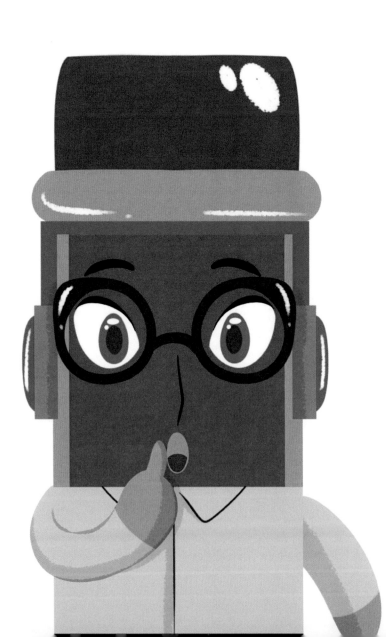

But Mike has a super, secretive, secret, a very BIG super, secretive, secret...

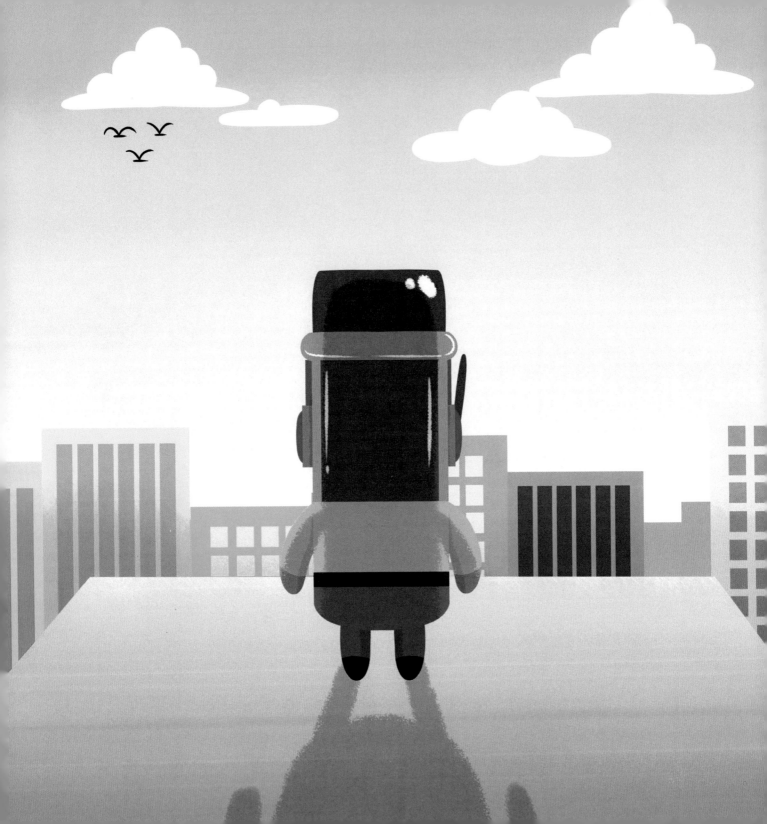

When Mike is not reading books from morning to night, hunting for new stories at the library, or spending time with Charlie, Mike uses his tremendous talents for...

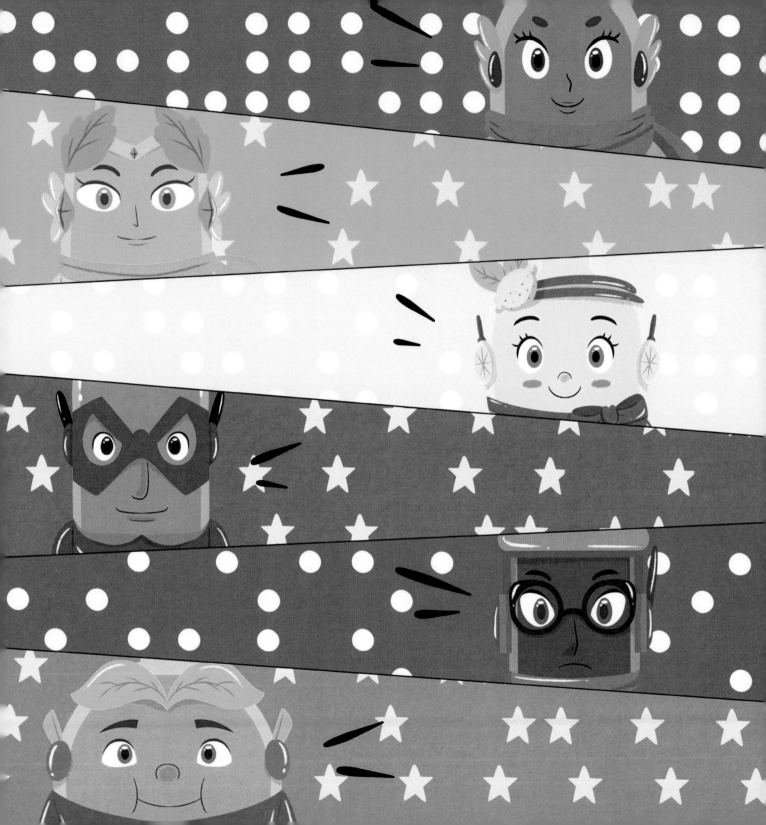

The Essential Heroes!!!

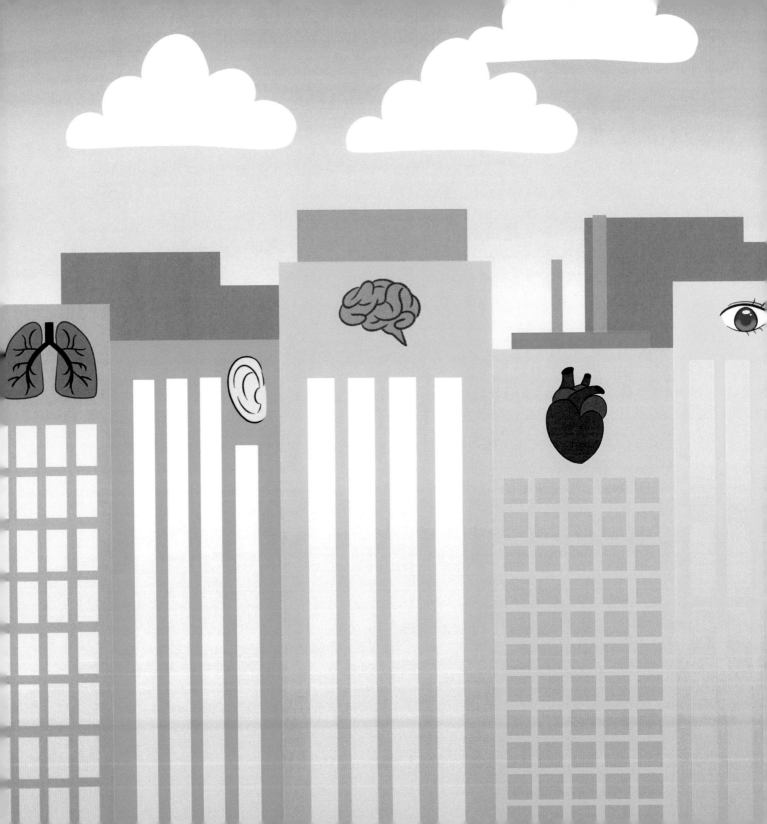

The Essential Heroes are a dedicated team of powerful friends that support Bodyville whenever there is a need!

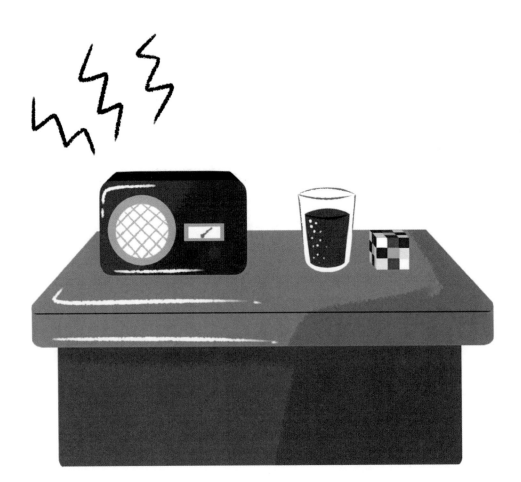

The Essential Heroes are called into action by Mr. Hypo. Mr. Hypo is the allusive and secret leader of the Essential Heroes. Mr. Hypo constantly watches over Bodyville, searching for anything and everything that needs hero help!

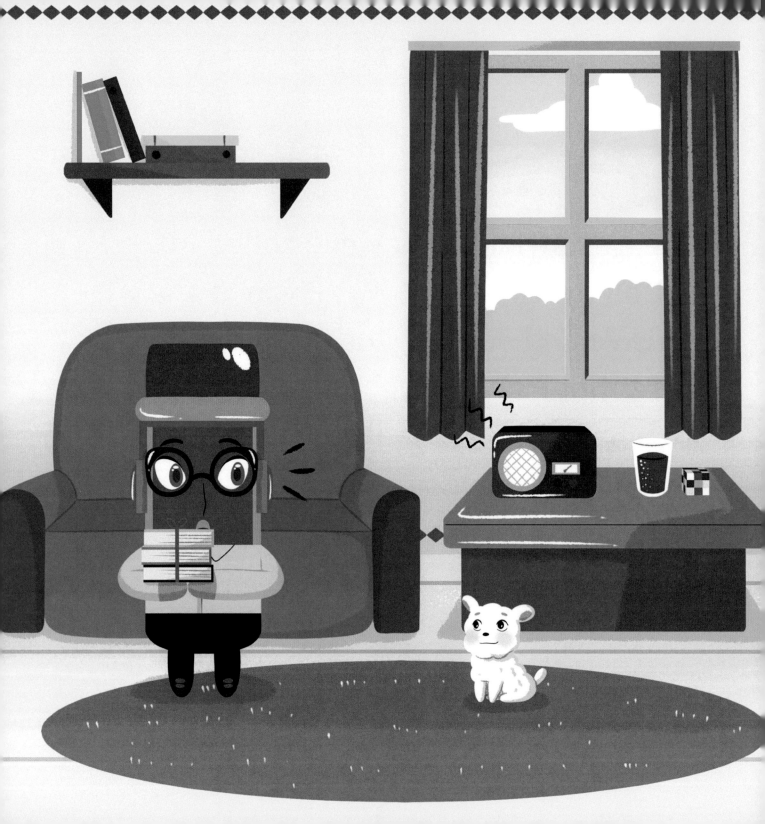

One day after coming back from a book-sale, Mike's super secret radio crackled to life causing Charlie to bark in excitement.

"This is Hypo calling Mike Melaleuca! I repeat, this is Hypo calling Mike Melaleuca! Come in Mike!"

"Mike Melaleuca here! Go ahead Mr. Hypo!"

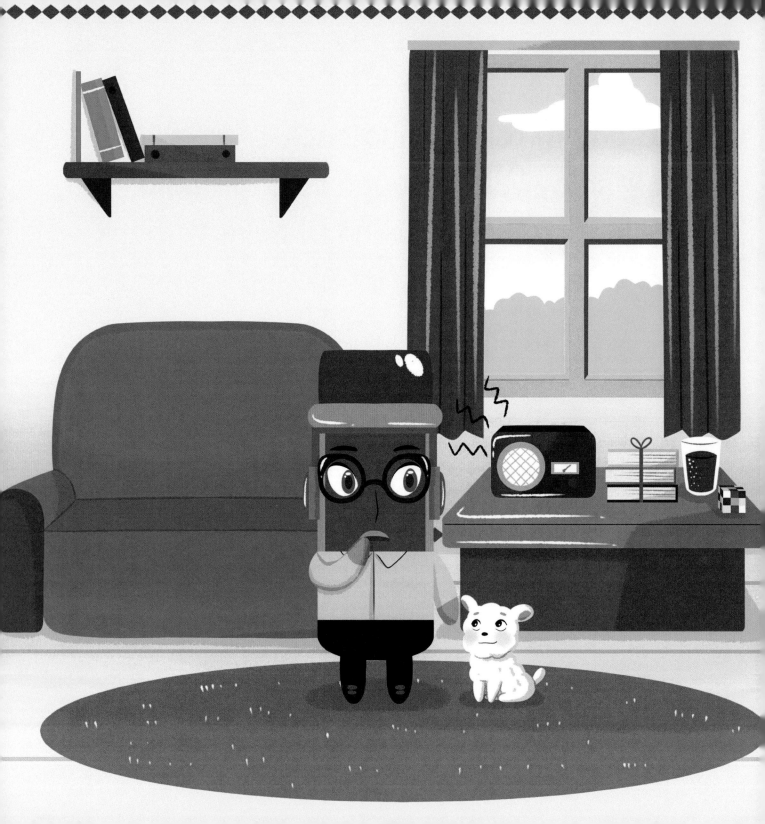

"Thank goodness we found you Mike!" said Hypo. "We just received word that Victor Virion has been spotted downtown."

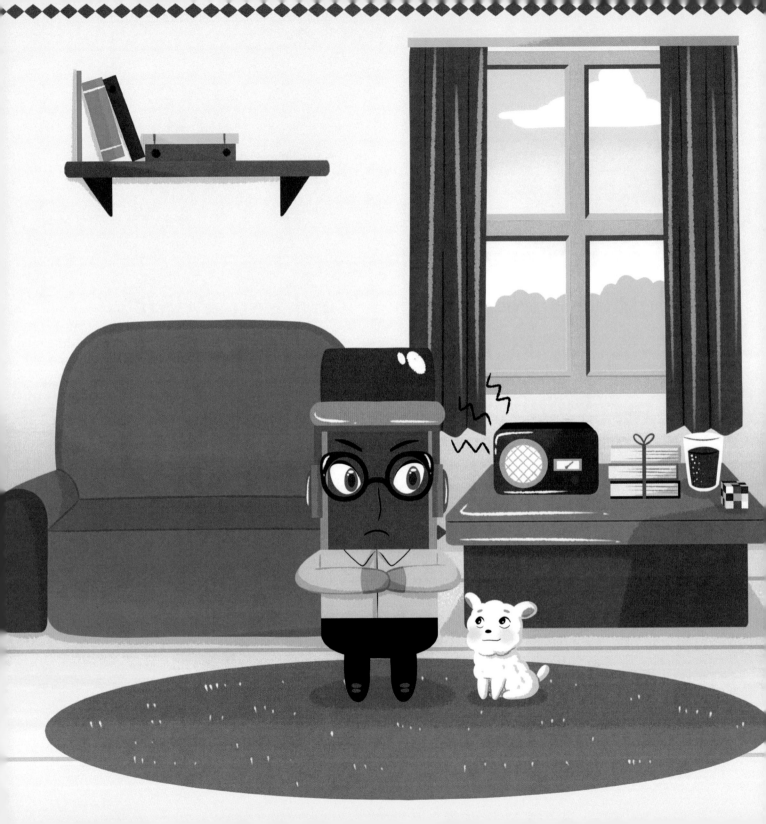

"Not Victor Virion," Mike said as he looked sadly at his stack of new books, knowing he wouldn't be reading them anytime soon.

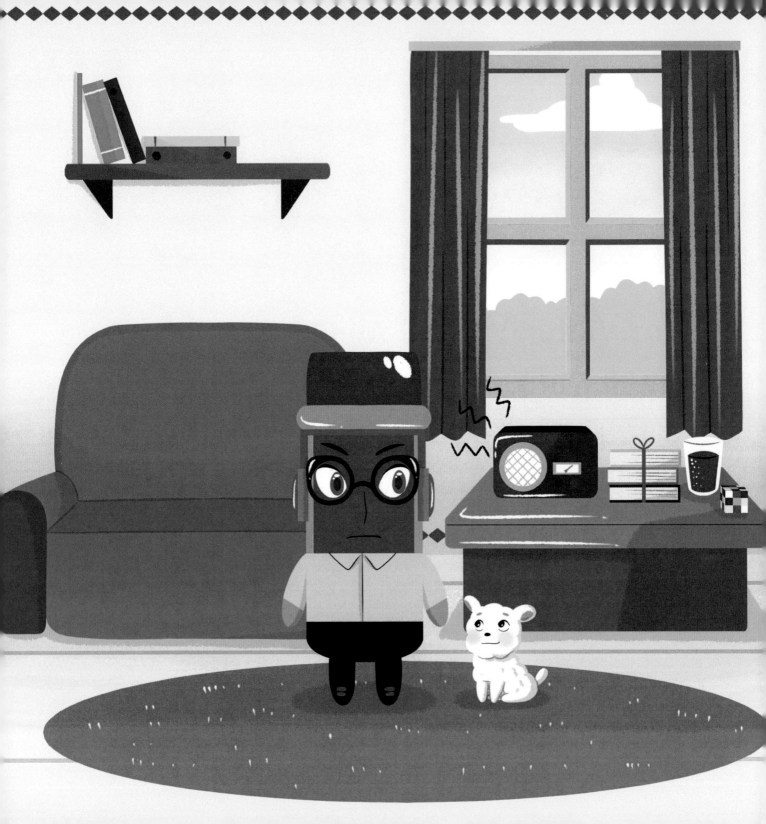

"Word on the street is, that he is planning on disrupting the Epidermis Festival!" Hypo said. "Can you stop him?"

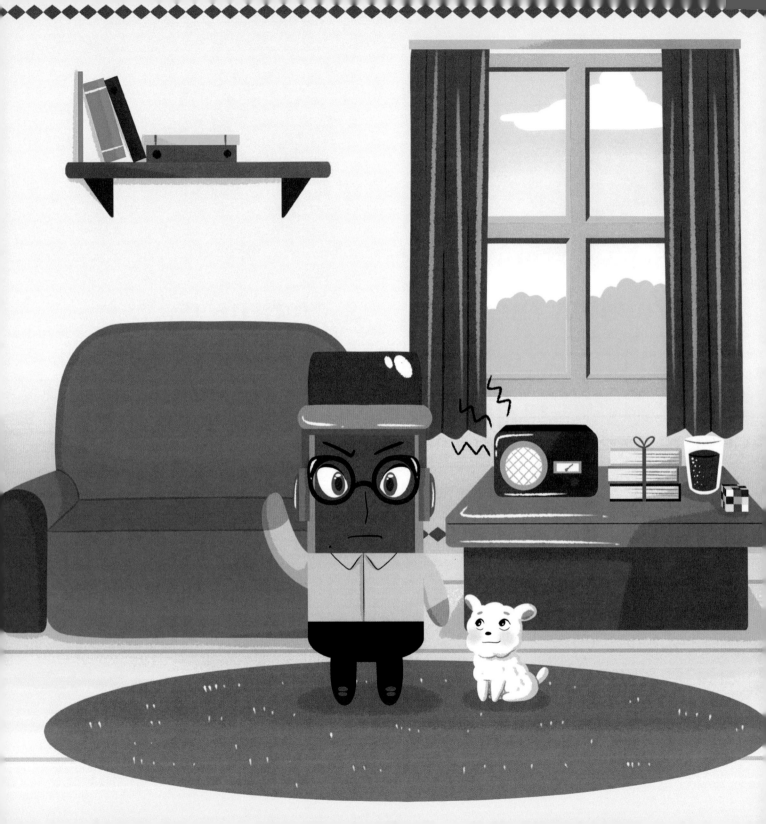

"I will do my best!" Mike said confidently. "If he gets to the festival, there is no telling what kind of damage he will cause!"

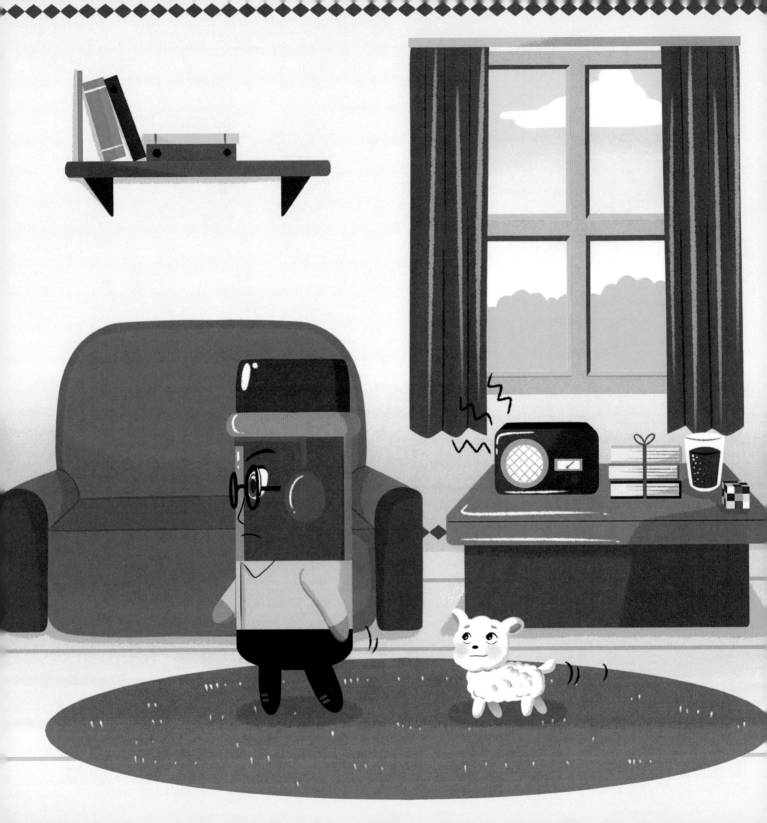

"Then hurry!" Hypo said passionately. "There is no time for delay! The festival has already started!"

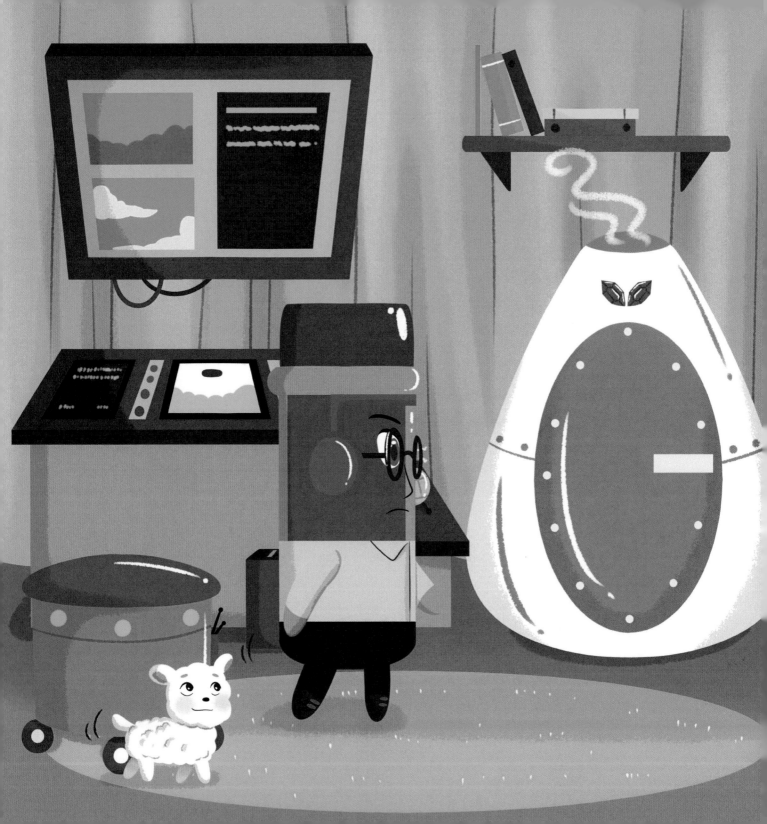

Charlie walked with Mike to his super secret diffuser room. The computer buzzed as the coordinates loaded.

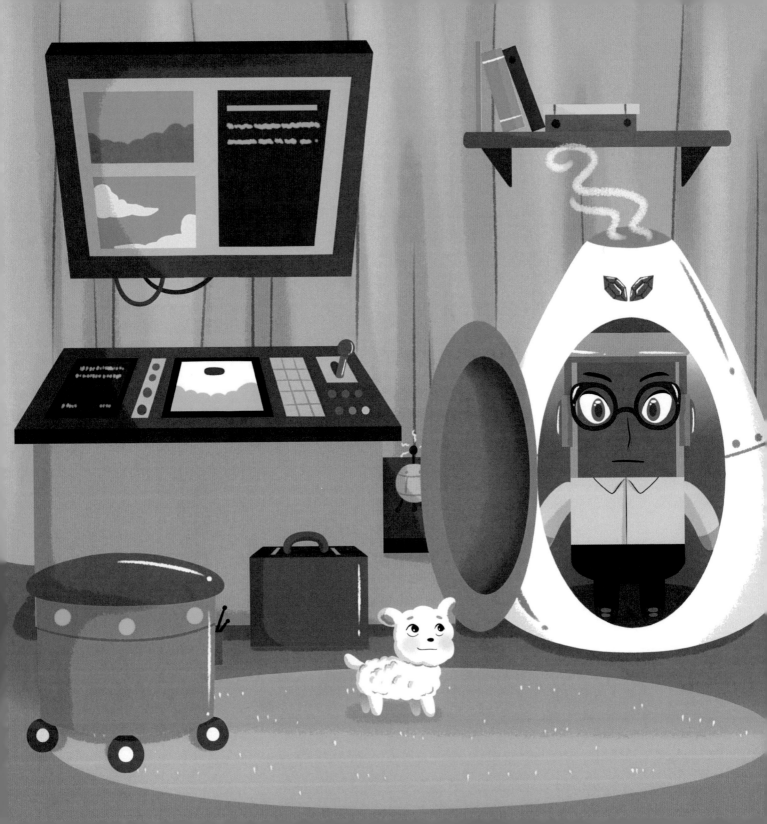

"We'll read our new stories when I get home tonight," Mike said to Charlie as he entered the diffuser and closed the door behind him. Mike took a deep breath and waited...

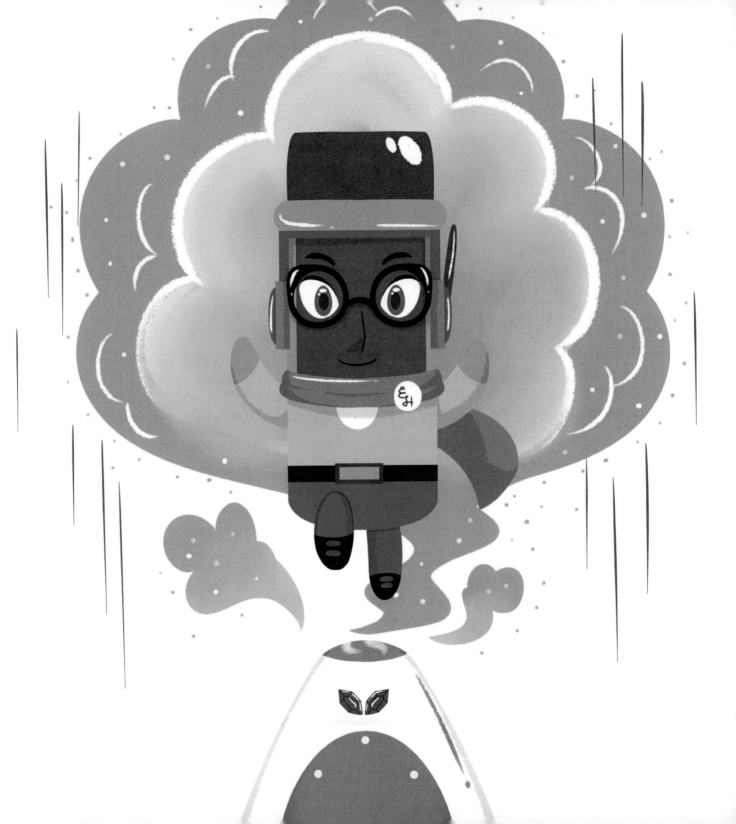

Mike burst out of the diffuser like a cannonball from a cannon! Up, up, up he flew until he was high enough to see all of Bodyville.

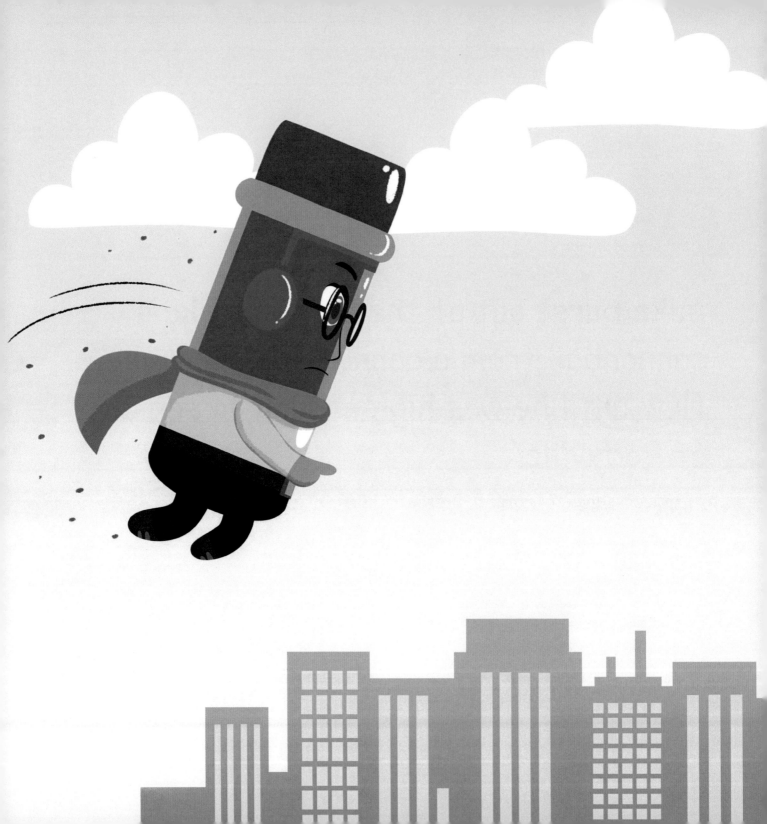

Being so high, it didn't take Mike long to spot the creepy, crawly, Victor Virion. Victor was making his way across town and toward the Epidermis Festival.

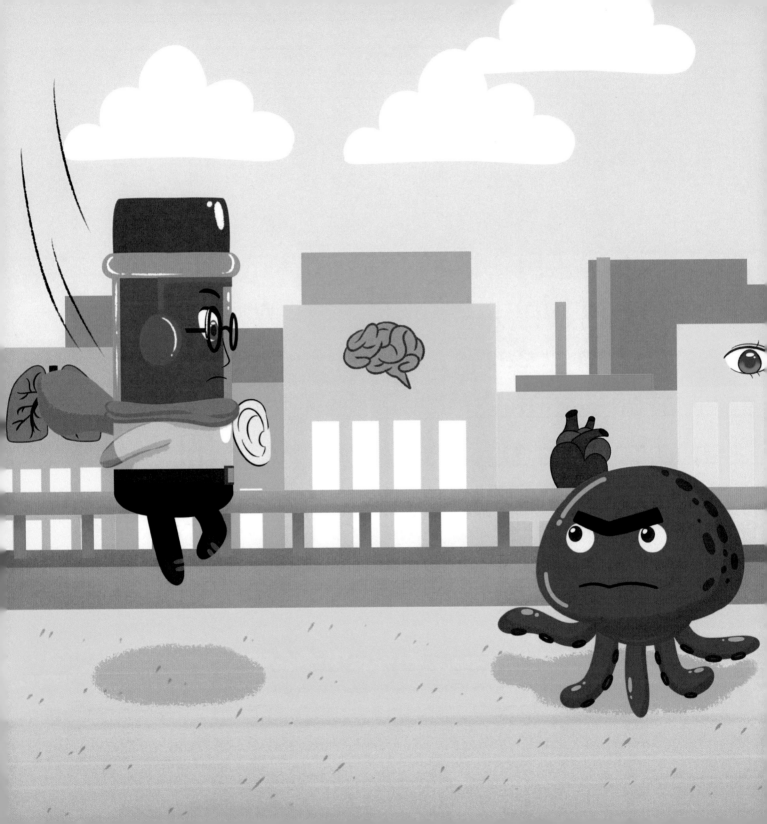

With a loud "thud," Mike landed in Victor's path. If Victor wanted to get to the festival, he was going to have to go through Mike first!

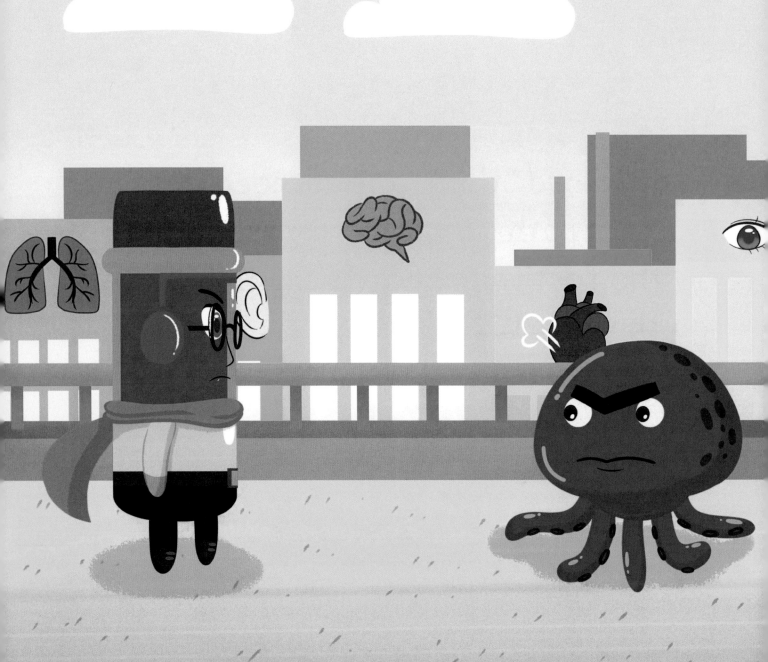

Victor inched nearer but Mike was ready for him. He had fought Victor before so he was prepared for Victor's tricks, or so he thought.

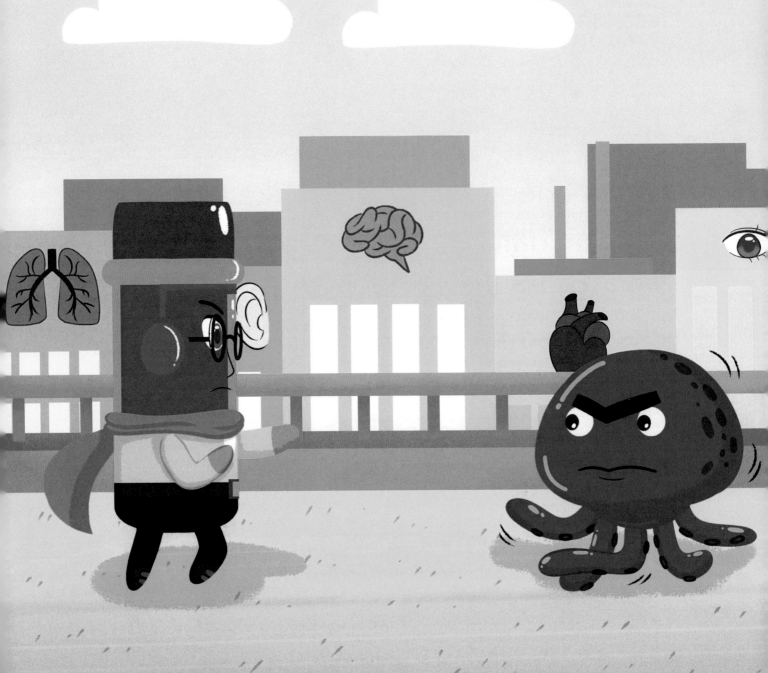

Victor squirmed his tentacled body nearer to Mike, preparing to strike. Mike raised his arms up, ready to block Victor's attack.

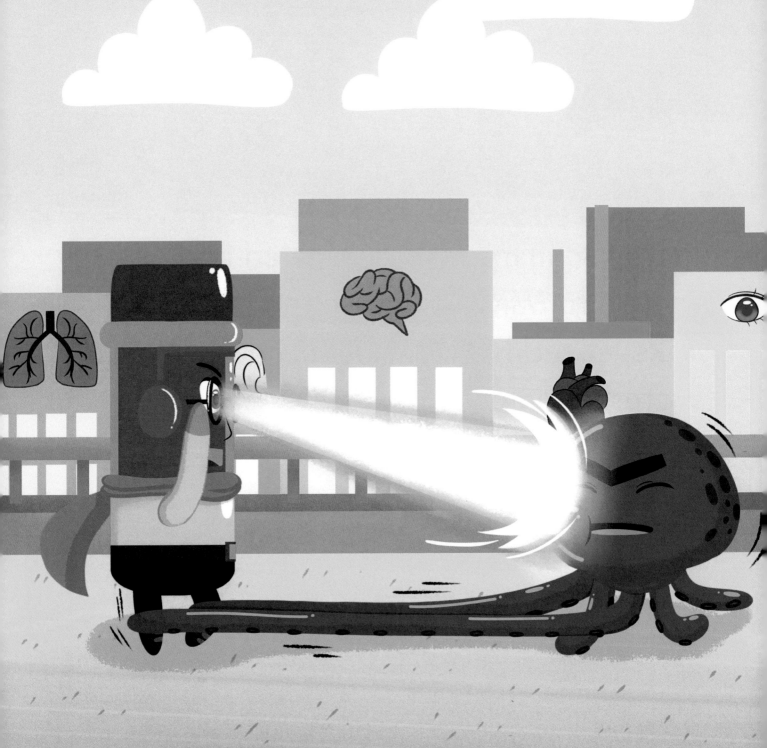

In the blink of an eye, Victor's two front tentacles shot toward Mike and grabbed his feet. Mike was ready for Victor's strike however and raised his hand to his powerful glasses releasing a blinding energy ray right back at Victor.

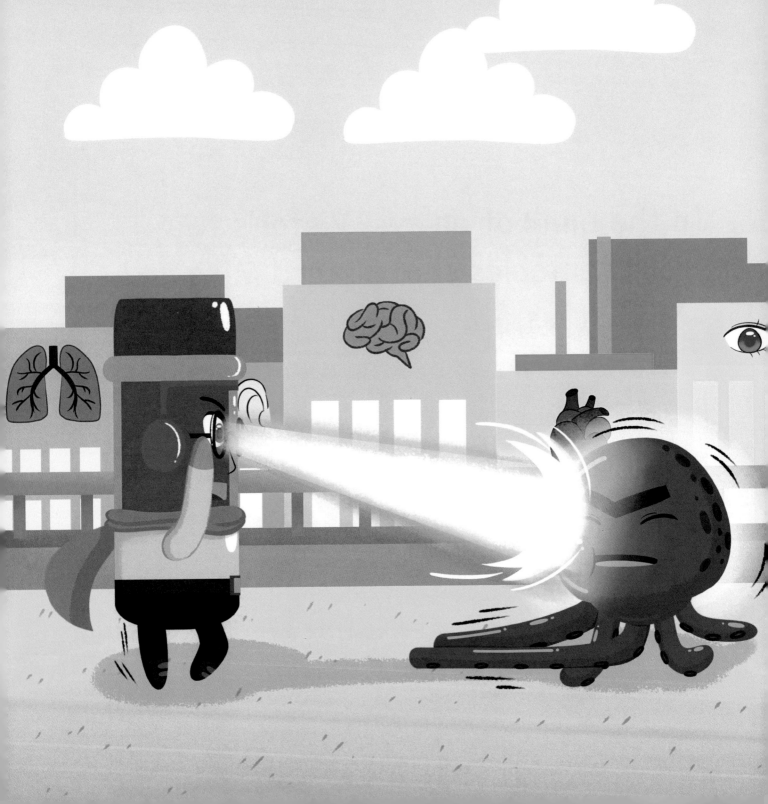

The ray of energy was too much for Victor to handle. He retracted his tentacles from Mike's feet and tried to get away but he couldn't. Mike's ray was too powerful.

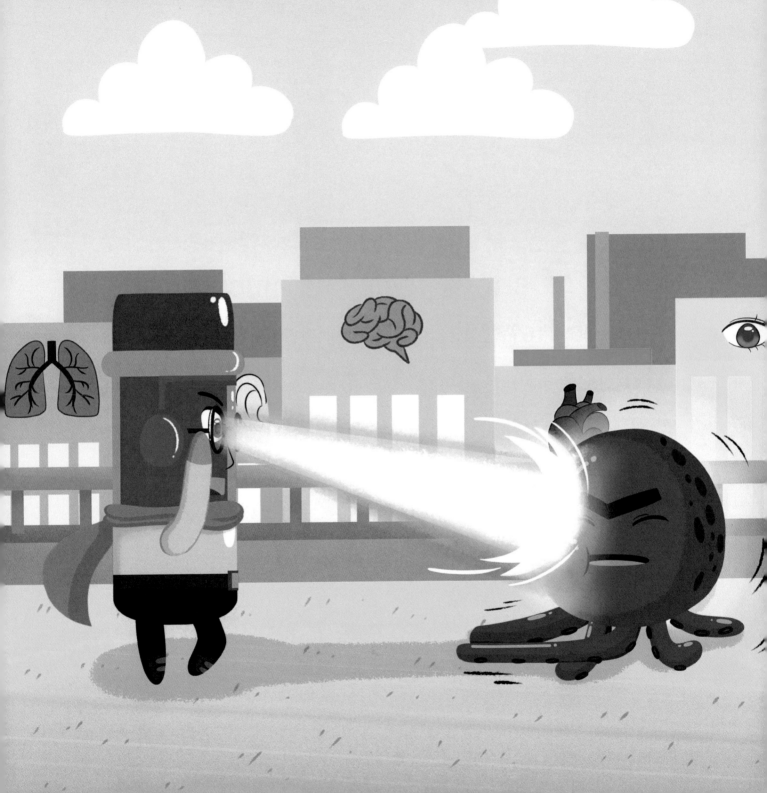

Mike took a step closer to Victor and kept beaming the energy ray into him. Every second Victor was exposed to it, his tentacles shrank until...

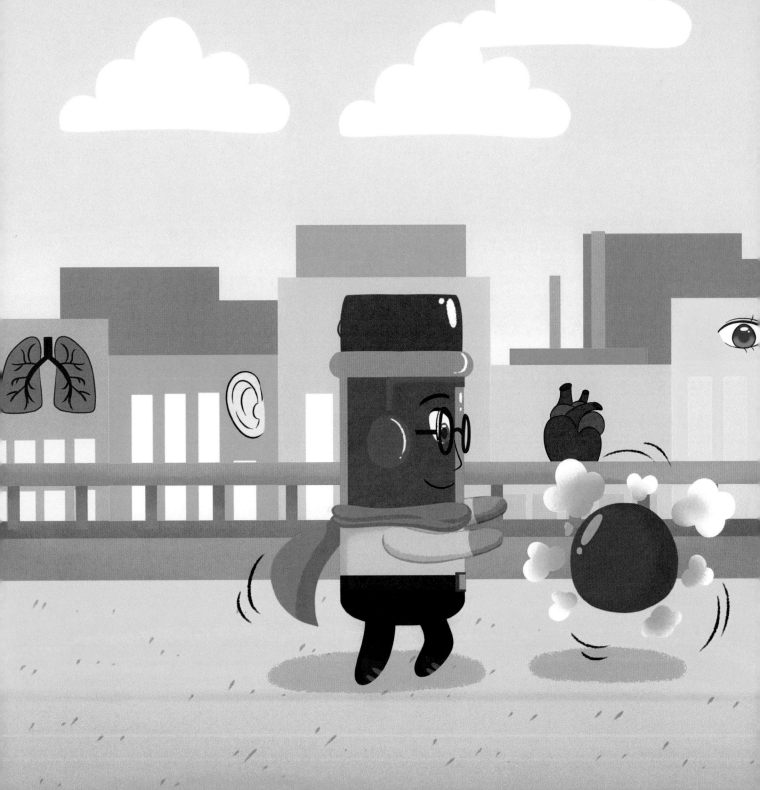

"Pop!" Victor had turned into a big, bouncy, ball. Mike smiled broadly as he reached for the ball. He had saved the Epidermis Festival and he now had a new toy for Charlie!

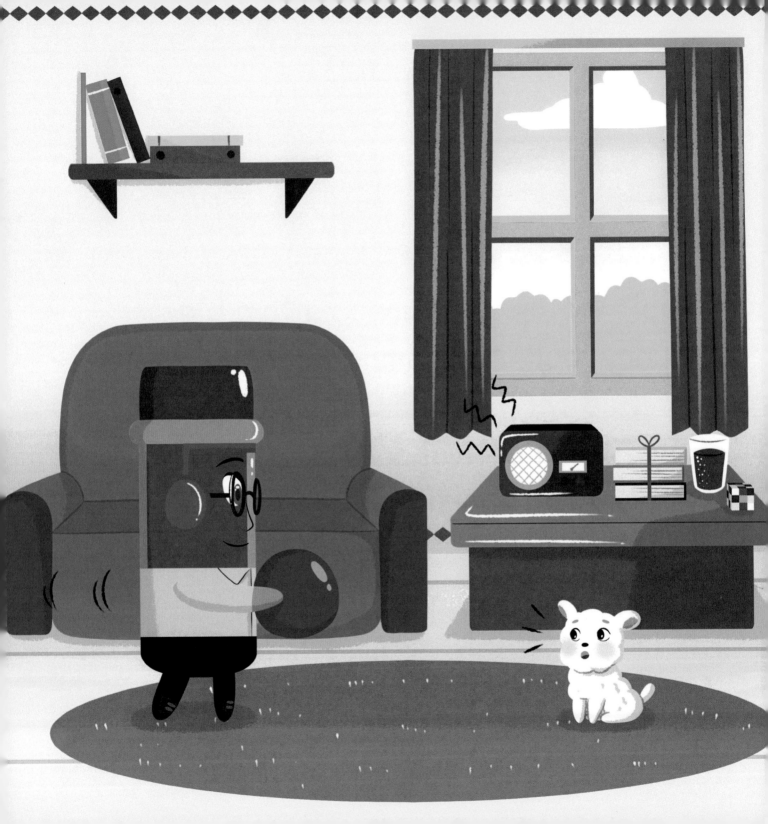

"Good work out there today," Hypo called out on the radio as Mike came home.

"Just doing my duty," Mike called back.

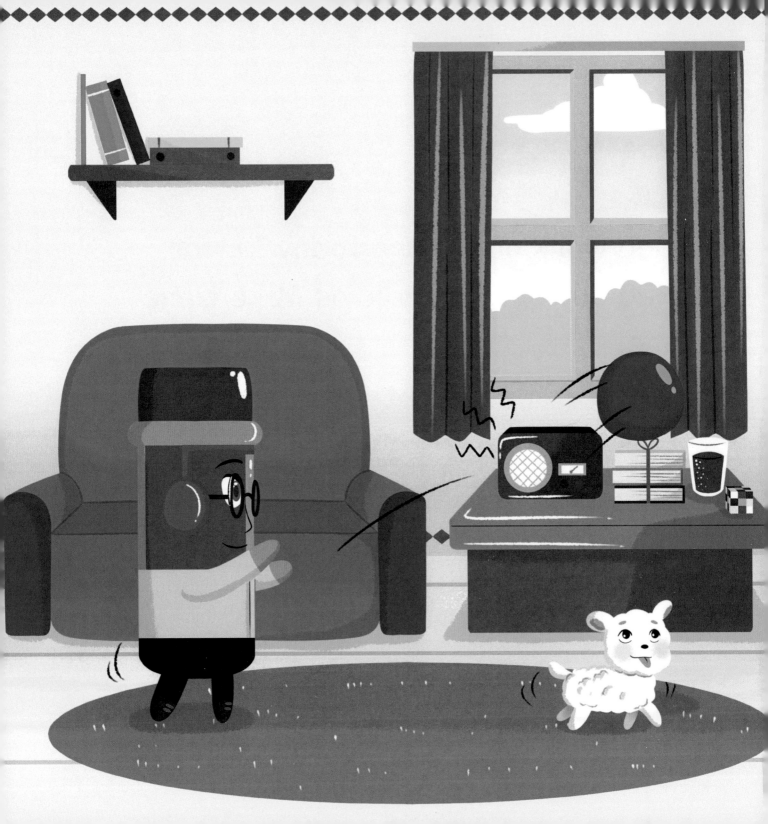

Mike tossed the ball up for Charlie who chased it into the next room.

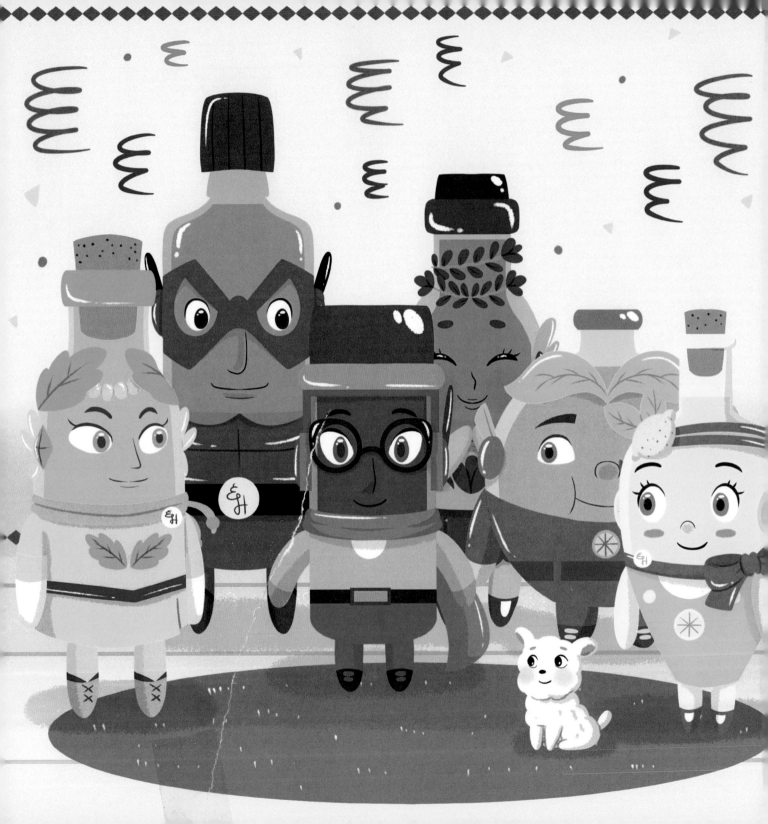

"Surprise!" all of Mike's friends called out as he entered the room. "You're a great member of the Essential Heroes!"

Mike beamed with happiness. Books, Charlie, and his best friends. What could be better?

Made in the
USA
Lexington, KY